ALZHEIMER'S

&

DEMENTIA

Paths to Take

By

Anne Elizabeth Nixon

Text copyright © 2016

By Anne Elizabeth Nixon

All Rights Reserved

As you go through life

savor the moments.

Enjoy them NOW!

You will never,

ever be sorry!

No one knows when

it may be too late.

DEDICATION

*I dedicate this book to Don, my loving husband,
and to all those who suffer
with this dreadful disease—
and to the caregivers who agonize in a way no
one else can fully appreciate.*

*We often blame ourselves, looking back on things
we've done or omitted,
wishing we could change them.
Keep those secrets to yourself, then forget them.*

*I get solace by thinking ahead
when we will be together again...*

PREFACE

My reason for this book is to give you as much help as I can, and I feel this is one way to accomplish that.

As I told you in my dedication, try your best not to blame yourself if you find, like I have, that you've "missed the mark" in your effort to do the right thing. I know it's difficult, but for your own health and that of your loved one, it is an important part of his or her care and yours. You need to be at your best to accomplish that.

Anne

CHAPTERS

1 – First Inkling, family history

2 – Looking back

3 – Diagnosis

4 – Medication

5 – Progression

6 – Changes, physical & mental

7 – Wandering

8 – Alert devices

9 – Memory care & paying for it

10 – Caregivers & agencies

11 – Today

Additional Comments

Additional Comments Two

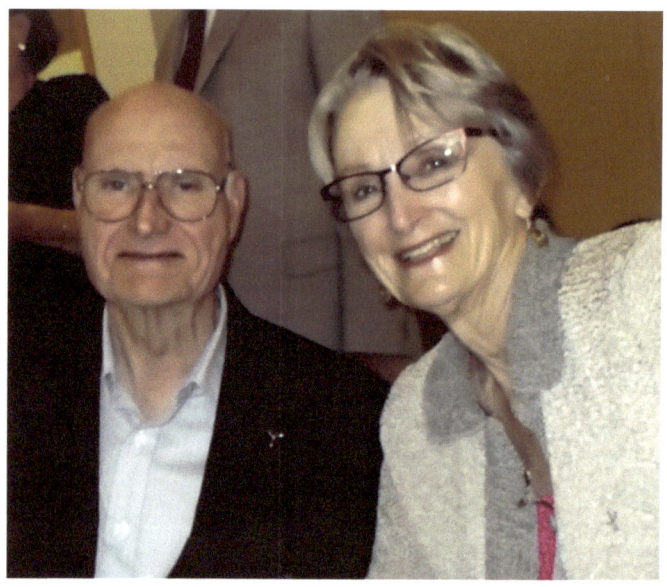

Don enjoyed this get-together of relatives, unaware it was a memorial service for a beloved relative.

CHAPTER ONE

First Inkling
Family History

Sometimes I wonder: is this a dream and I'm going to wake up to find everything is back to normal?
Then reality returns with a feeling that's impossible to describe.

Of all the diseases that might have befallen my husband, dementia and eventually Alzheimer's were farthest from what might have come to mind. In the 35 years we were married, until he began medications for this disease, he'd never taken pills. While others spoke of aches and pains, a bum knee or arthritic hip, Don had nothing in common with them.

We both loved to laugh and his sense of humor was the driving force of his personality. As an outside salesman for machinery, his customers trusted and enjoyed him. I can only imagine how they looked forward to upbeat chats when he called on them.

At a class reunion I learned about his good memory when he was in high school. "He always remembered everything," a friend recalled.
"Guess I took after Mom," Don told his old pal, winking. And it was true. I'd already discovered Bess had a fabulous way of recalling not only names and places, but when something had happened.

We spent ten years as full-time RVers, and at one point became interested in Civil War battlefields. Generals' names, the number of troops, and details of those battles were thrown at us day after day. I felt inundated in facts. But my husband took it all in. After we settled down a few years later friends and relatives were often interested and asked us questions.

I could only sputter, "Gee, I don't remember," while Don came up with the answers easily.

Earlier traits may indicate nothing about what is to follow later.

We'd both had difficult first marriages and when we met in a singles' group in our mid-forties, we recognized how much we were interested in the same things. So our relationship was easy-going and happy and funny and very loving.

One morning about 20 years into our marriage Don unleashed words so unusual to him, my surprise led me to say, "If you had acted like that when I first met you I wouldn't have been interested in getting to know you better." In those few moments we'd both said something neither of us had ever voiced before—because no two people could ever have enjoyed each other more! He stared at me and I at him: where had that come from, I'm sure we must have been wondering. Only I'm sure his thoughts were sprinkled with some @#$%&!

I was in the midst of taking over the writing of our family history from a cousin who could no longer finish it, and spent early afternoons working on that while Don golfed a few blocks away. Eight or ten men got together every morning at 11:00 to play nine holes—rain, hail, sleet, snow, or sunshine, and one day all of those. They knew each other well and enjoyed the exercise and companionship. At about 2 PM Don returned home, and I'd hear his happy call to me from the other end of the house. As we enjoyed a snack or lunch, he filled me in on local news, and I discovered men and women gossip with equal interest. But interspersed in his tales to me were never, ever unkind words about anyone.

I must make it clear to you that it isn't what a person says that screams alarm, but the change from their normal behavior.

After my father-in-law was widowed in a small Midwest town his family and friends worried about him because it seemed he'd forgotten how to get around town in his car. "He seemed not to know the way to places he'd gone to for years," a friend told us.

We flew back to get him, and in his car we all drove out to the west coast. Don sold Pop's Chevrolet with his approval even though we noticed no disorientation around home. But when he fell on our gravel road and hit his head, our doctor prescribed a medication and told us he must never be left alone. That meant it was necessary for him to live in an assisted care home near us. Pop played by ear any instrument you placed in his hands, and entertained them all with his guitar and harmonica and singing. Because of his outgoing personality and gift of music, I saw him as the fun-loving man he'd always been.

However, when Don and I talked to one of the caregivers who had worked in the home where Pop lived, we heard, "Don seems to be following in his father's footsteps, doesn't he?"

I was surprised to hear her words, for I'd never thought of Pop as having had dementia. But caregivers know their people in ways we never can, so possibly Don had that dread disease in genes that were handed down from one generation to another.

Just because there might be a family history of this disease doesn't mean it will continue on in future generations.

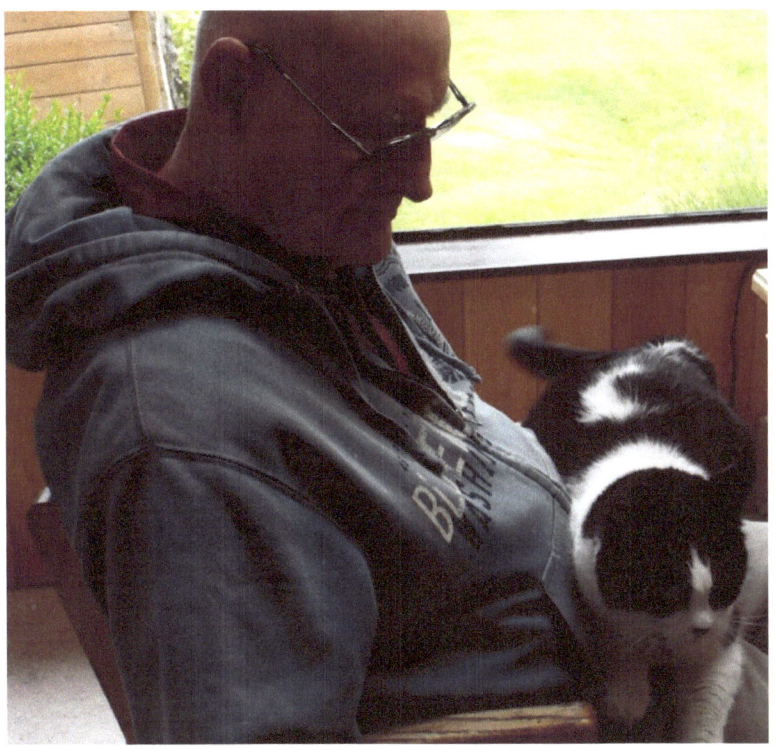

Animals can make wonderful pals for those with dementia and Alzheimer's disease. As time went on, however, his kitties were less responsive when he became more heavy-handed.

CHAPTER TWO

Looking Back

As I search for my discovery of Don's Alzheimer's, I find nothing. My husband found it himself.

"Sometimes I feel confused," he told me one afternoon.

How I responded I don't remember. But we were in our sixties, and aging is inevitable. Maybe we'd like to scream, "I want to stay young. I demand it!" but we can't.

Don didn't pursue his complaint, and I forgot about it because it didn't seem serious. Another reason I decided it was nothing to worry about was because I'd heard that the person himself never knows when he has Alzheimer's disease. That was the determining factor, my information touted. "If you know there's something the matter, it isn't." So obviously, I remember thinking, everything is okay. That was that, and I was satisfied—and relieved.

Then one day the phone rang and one of his golf buddies said, "Tell Don we'll meet at 10:00 today, will you?"

"Why so early?" I wondered, and was told, "There's a kids' tournament later, so we have to get moving."

But I couldn't let it go, for it was almost the time he was to be there. So finally I got the real answer. "Well, Don's so slow these days he always arrives late. So we've decided to tell him half an hour early from now on."

What????

We spoke a bit longer, and I remember the fear I felt tightening in my chest. Arrives late? He never left the house late. What was he doing? It seemed he was fiddling around at his car as he got out his clubs.

Why????

I told him the earlier time and hoped all would go well. His friends helped him, and as time went on he needed it more and more. No one alerted me, and either I was unaware the problem was increasing or I was afraid to look into it. On Tuesdays we met friends at the Moose lodge for tacos, some of them fellow golfers. When Don gave money to a pal to pay for his and my tacos I didn't know of it for many months; my job was to head into the bar to get beers and colas. When I came back balancing the drinks for us and others on a tray, I didn't see anything awry. No one purposely hid Don's confusion, for again, I think they probably thought I knew.

At home he seemed no different. He kept our big yard mowed and trimmed, his cat following him until the wheelbarrow was full, and then jumping up on top of limbs and scraps to ride to the dumping pile with Don. We often laughed at his little pal, and if animals can sense illness, his kitty didn't give any hint of trouble. When we had our fun-loving friends and large family over Don joked and chatted, and helped me by serving cocktails and wine. There simply was nothing that alerted me. Whether it worried him, I will never know, for he didn't speak of it other than his saying he'd felt confused many months earlier.

One Thanksgiving we were all together at our house for dinner. Don took drink orders as we sat in the living room, and soon he and a cousin were delivering them. At the table one lady had trouble, spilling food onto her lap and finally on the floor. She'd obviously had too much to drink, very unlike her. Until she mentioned it a few months later I thought maybe she'd gulped it down rather than sipped. "That was an awfully strong drink Don made for me," she said. "I'm so sorry I got food on your carpet."
That seemed odd, for he hated over-strong drinks himself and I'd always enjoyed his bartending. Looking back, though, it could have been a warning.

He must have realized his strength was waning, for he began using his strongest golf club, unlike his usual way. The first sign was when his driver head broke off from the shaft. He got it fixed and nothing more was said. The second thing was that I noticed he wasn't hitting as far on days when I played with him. But again, we were aging like all folks do. The third clue was my seeing him hit fairway shots with his driver. I hadn't known why the club had broken until much later, and now I remember saying, "Why aren't you using your fairway clubs?" His answer was, "If I want to win money (the fellows put in money and divvied up later in the clubhouse), I gotta use this." And then fourth, the driver broke again. This time it was unfixable and he bought a new club.

Eventually he quit playing golf with the men and I knew he couldn't keep up any more; he'd been diagnosed with dementia by then. We'd head for the driving range where he hit a bucket of balls, sometimes very well and other times like a beginner. But he was outdoors and at the golf course, both things he loved. About that same time he began riding with me as I played with the ladies' club, and he came along to monthly meetings. He sat on the couch watching the golf channel on TV, and every so often he might get up to see that I was still close by. I'd wave to him and that satisfied his apprehension.

Out on the course, however, there were occasional outbursts and I'd say, "If you can't be quiet while the gals play you can't come with me." Those words and a scowl were usually enough to quiet him, but soon it would happen again. It began with enjoying to ride along and progressed to a jealousy or despair at not being able to play. Sometimes I thought it was the latter, for once he got out of the cart and took one of my clubs so he could hit a ball. I had to explain it was time for only ladies to play and he could hit balls later.

When we began playing couples' golf on Sundays I always paired up with friends. Don had golfed with the husband in the past and was always very glad to see him. Score never mattered much on Sundays, so when his pal said, "Don, why don't you take one of Anne's clubs and hit a ball or two," there was no one to object. I appreciated the man's thoughtfulness as much as my husband did! That continued until I had to quit playing because of my health, and then it became a fading memory.

Core muscles are those in the abdominal region, low back, and up to the diaphragm. Don began experiencing a lessening of strength.

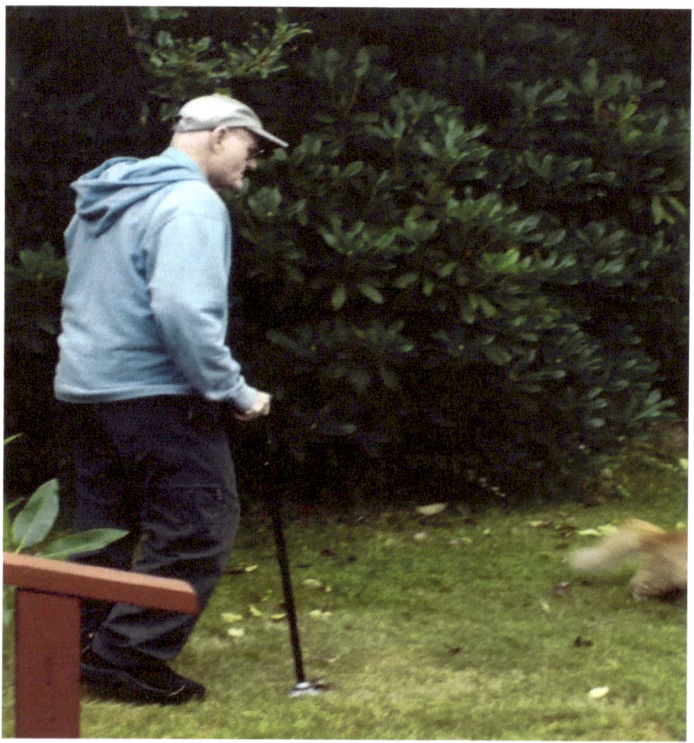

I bought him a cane so he could go into the uneven yard by himself and take his kitties for walks.

CHAPTER THREE

Diagnosis

I can't remember what brought us to the point of going to the doctor. But I wasn't concerned we might be learning that he had any disease. Don was the healthiest human being I'd ever known. When I first met him he had his wisdom teeth removed and swallowed blood, causing him to vomit. Twenty-five years later there had been two days of flu-like illness, but until that time he'd never been sick. It was as though his body had declared, I refuse to waste time with illness!

So that morning when the doctor asked me to come in as he saw Don, I went without suspecting anything. We sat in the examining room together as the doctor turned to pull out a sheet of paper. He had some questions he wanted to ask, he explained.

"Name five animals for me, Don." But he didn't know the answers. What, I thought? Am I hearing things? Those were questions for a young child! My husband hesitated and glanced over at me. "Go ahead," I prompted. This all sounded silly and I began telling myself the animals—cows, horses, goats, cats, dogs…" But Don sat there, eventually saying possibly one animal or two, but no others. So the doctor asked another question from the paper. No answer at all.

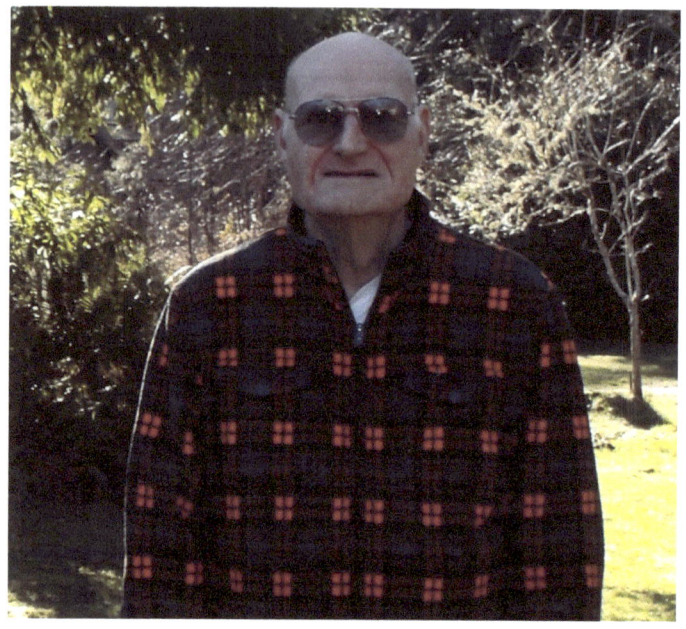

For a person who enjoyed the outdoors like Don, it was important that he spend as much time as weather allowed out in the yard or on the deck.

By this time I had become worried. Was he nervous? Why hadn't he spit out the answers he knew so easily?

"I think we'll schedule you for an x-ray, Don," the doctor told him. He tried to sound casual so as not to worry his patient, but he knew me well enough to know I had great concern. I'd never been a worrier, but waiting for the doctor's call left me with a heavy heart, suspecting the brain scan would be abnormal in some way.

A week later I got the results. *And that's when my world fell apart!*

Don may never have realized how serious his condition was. If he did, he never talked about it. And, not wanting to worry him, neither did I. We went on as we had before, but not as we had before either, for that was on the surface, and he had a disease that was worsening. I felt a sadness that couldn't be brushed aside.

Eventually I ordered a book called "Alzheimer's Disease" from the Mayo Clinic, and sat down to read it from cover to cover. But after the first dozen pages I closed it and never read another word. I wish I had studied those chapters so I'd have known what to expect. But my heart was broken, and I felt I couldn't face the months and years ahead if I knew what those doctors were going to tell me. That was a serious mistake, however, and that's why I'm writing this short book—so you will know what you might do to make life better and easier. Just because Don had certain symptoms doesn't mean your loved one will, but the general pathway can prepare you. I wish I had been able to spot many things that I missed. I'm convinced it would have helped us both.

Becoming a Power of Attorney (POA) for the ill person is an extremely important step. You can then make necessary decisions in his or her behalf.

There are two ways to do this:

1 - You can have an attorney draw up those papers and you sign before him.

2 - The least expensive way is to call your nearest hospital and ask if they have the form for becoming a person's power of attorney. Fill it out in the presence of two witnesses and have it notarized.

Be very sure to do this!

The Alzheimer Association says this: "Alzheimer's disease is a progressive brain disorder that damages and eventually destroys brain cells, leading to memory loss and changes in thinking and other brain functions. It usually develops slowly and gradually gets worse as brain function declines and brain cells eventually wither and die. Ultimately, Alzheimer's is fatal, and currently, there is no cure."

CHAPTER FOUR

Medication

Our doctor moved to another state before any treatment began. The physician taking over his practice told me, "There's a medication we could start Don on—"

"Yes. Right now, let's start," I interrupted.

So Aricept, 10 mg twice a day was prescribed. He explained there were other medications that he could add, but nothing to begin at that time. Unfortunately, even though I had worked in doctors' offices my entire working life, I didn't question him about that, probably because I felt so shocked and at loose ends about this disease. I'm not sure if it might have made any difference, but looking back now, I believe it would not.

Eventually Don began taking Namenda, 10 mg twice a day also.

After being on those two for several months he seemed to be better, I thought.

That Christmas we traveled to California to be with our family for the holiday. One very good friend with whom I had worked, asked if I'd like Don to be seen by the doctor she worked for. He was an excellent diagnostician, she said.

After a lengthier examination than he'd had by the new doctor at home, this physician suggested trying the Exelon patch, in addition to the other two. But what helps one person doesn't necessarily help another, so after a lengthy trial he determined it should be stopped.

Pharmaceutical companies are very good about helping those who have a hard time paying for medications. If you feel the need, ask if they have a program to subsidize or suspend all cost for months or years. There's no reason to feel shy about this.

And there is a Canadian pharmacy called Planet Drugs Direct that sells medications in the United States. They are manufactured in the United Kingdom and other European and Asian countries. It is a great help for the very high cost of dementia drugs. Any time you find a less expensive generic medication, or ones from a foreign country, check with your pharmacist to see if they will be equal to the brand name pills or those manufactured in the United States. He can tell you.

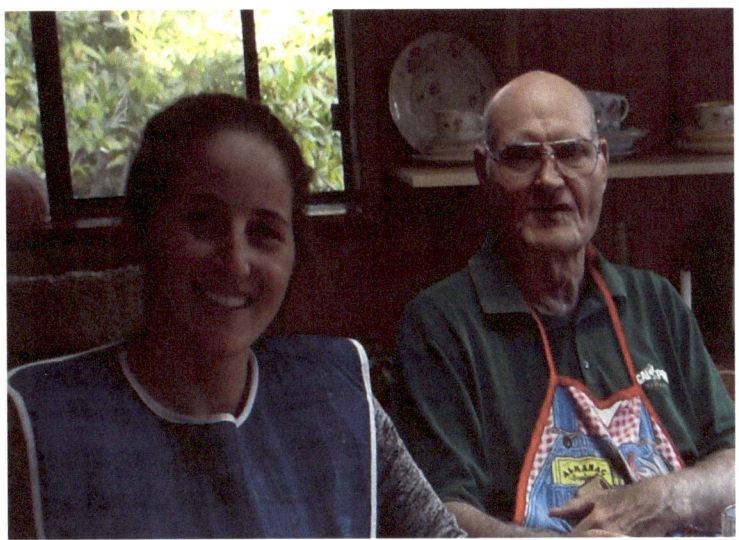

This photo was taken with his granddaughter. He enjoyed her company so much!

The California doctor referred Don to a hematologist since his laboratory tests had shown he was anemic. But there was nothing to be done about that, he said, and iron tablets or shots would not help in his case. This, however, may have had nothing to do with his dementia.

There is a condition of the brain that can be dramatically cured with a shunt or drain, called hydrocephalus (water on the brain). The referral to a neurosurgeon led to Don being prepped for a look-see. I prayed the doctor would find that was his problem, that he'd be well again. I was waiting for the neurosurgeon to come out and tell me, "All's well. I was successful."

But it was not to be.

One day I found a "cure for Alzheimer's disease" on the internet. Way deep inside I must have known better, but I read the promise. It said certain vegetables and fruits, a nap, and something else I can't remember now, would make the person suffering with this horrible disease well. In just a few weeks, it claimed, I'd notice a difference. Because doctors were so jealous of his brilliant finding, he warned, his cure might be forced from the internet. **(See last chapter re this)**

Oddly, I fell for this, and probably the reason was that I so desperately wanted to see a cure. But, broken-hearted, I stopped that diet, knowing I'd been duped like probably hundreds or maybe thousands. Before discontinuing that regimen I'd stopped his Namenda and Aricept so I could evaluate the change, and had to begin it again. I found him happier and enjoying life as he hadn't on the medications. But I didn't know what that meant, so I felt I had to start it again.

I remember the disgust I felt for anyone who treated his fellow human beings this way.

Some people become aggressive, which Don did occasionally. Our doctor prescribed an easy-to-tolerate medication, Gabapentin, and that helped for a while. But eventually it worked in the opposite way, and had to be discontinued.

Later, by another doctor, he was given Depakote in a very high dosage for the same symptom, aggression. While Don tolerated medicine well, that was way, way too much. Consequently, he fell one day and hit his head, and then a day or so later became dizzy, ending up in the Emergency Room twice. As his POA (power of attorney) I asked the dose be reduced, and finally discontinued. You know your loved one best, and you must be pro-active in his or her care. Don't hesitate to speak up when you can see medicine is harmful, or not helping with the cause for which it was given in the first place.

You have now become the patient's eyes and ears, and it is important you remember that. I cannot stress this enough!

Aggression among males with female (or male) caregivers is not new or unusual, I understand. Particularly, Don was not happy when being helped in the bathroom by women. But aggression can't be tolerated when it becomes hurtful, and when he grabbed a caregiver's hand or shoulder, that was over the line. The drug given must fit the "crime," however. This aggression began when we first hired an in-home caregiver after I injured my knee, and it continued to his memory care home.

A study done by the University of Michigan and Johns Hopkins reveals a *strategy to minimize the use of drugs for behavior problems*, dubbed DICE—describe, investigate, create and evaluate. This data has been collected from two decades of research studies. The name of the article I read was called, "Easing the Behavior Problems of Alzheimer's without Drugs." I warned that a patient must never be slammed with a huge dose of a strong medication! *This was done twice* to Don by the same doctor and without telling me! Both times I *fought a battle* for decreasing the dosage, then discontinuing it—and won after many phone calls.

When Don fell and struck his head after taking those very strong pills for aggression, he was forced to use a wheelchair. A while later, after it had been stopped, I asked the caregivers if he could be helped to walk for a short time daily, hopefully getting back on his feet again. They helped him into the dining room, using a walker. I didn't reverse my thoughts about him walking, but I feared he might fall and be worse off than before.

As I struggled to do the right thing for Don, I asked to talk to the memory care community's director. When she heard I wanted to talk about his medical care, she thought it best for me to talk to the nurse. The nurse and I sat down together with a notebook in which his medications were detailed for each day, strength, how much taken, when begun and when discontinued. Then we began talking about his walking.

"I think it would be wise to call Don's doctor and request a physical therapy evaluation. That could tell us whether it's possible to get his strength back for walking." I agreed that was a good idea and I called to set it up.

It would all be done at his memory care home, both evaluation and the physical therapy sessions, which were recommended. Nothing much came of this because no one took the time to help him use the walker except early in the morning when a couple of caregivers got him up. Don's being afraid of falling made it difficult.

Keep a close eye on your loved one's medication and behavior.

There is a new drug for Alzheimer's disease at this time, one that was approved by the FDA on July 13, 2023. The name is LEQEMBI, and it slows the symptoms. The cost and accessibility is unknown now, but be sure to look into something so important!

CHAPTER FIVE

Progression

Observing the disabilities of people with dementia and Alzheimer's, which is one of the many forms of dementia, you'll discover there is great variety. It depends on which areas of the brain are affected.

One of Don's difficulties became speech. When we were with friends he began putting a hand in front of his mouth and speaking more quietly. "Speak up," someone might growl, which, as it seemed to bother him, hurt me. I remember once lashing out, saying, "Leave him alone." That was not like him. One joke had always reminded him of another, but now that fun-loving attitude was changing, little by little.

And as music started for dancing, I became the one who urged him onto the dance floor. We'd always loved to dance and his reluctance puzzled me.

Driving became one of the first problems for a friend of ours, and soon the spouse was the sole driver. But that was a later difficulty for Don. One day he failed to stop for a policeman after not getting in the correct lane; he had no answer for the questions the cop asked. I tried to answer for him.

"It seems your husband has a problem understanding," he told me, then walked around the car to speak to me. "I think you should take him to an emergency room. He may have had a small stroke." Then he walked back to the driver's side window and calmly said, "Open your door and get out, sir. I want you to change places with your wife." When there was no action or answer, the policeman opened the door and ordered him out. I drove home. That was the end of his driving unless I was with him in our very rural community. If he was simply going a short distance where there were few cars and one lane I rode with him for another month.

***I didn't suspect**. Those words were a common thread as I look back upon our life at that time. **He had never done or acted like that before**, were others.*

So, if it's worrisome or unusual or just gives you an uneasy feeling, don't simply let it slide by. Investigate. Speaking with self-consciousness and reluctance getting up to dance doesn't warrant investigation right away. But becoming a poor driver does. It's your responsibility.

Alzheimer's disease is so frightening that it changes us along with the one suffering that illness.

Taking a privilege away is difficult at best. And getting rid of a car is often extremely so. I know of a woman who fought it until her children had to lie by telling her they were taking it to be repaired for something that didn't exist.

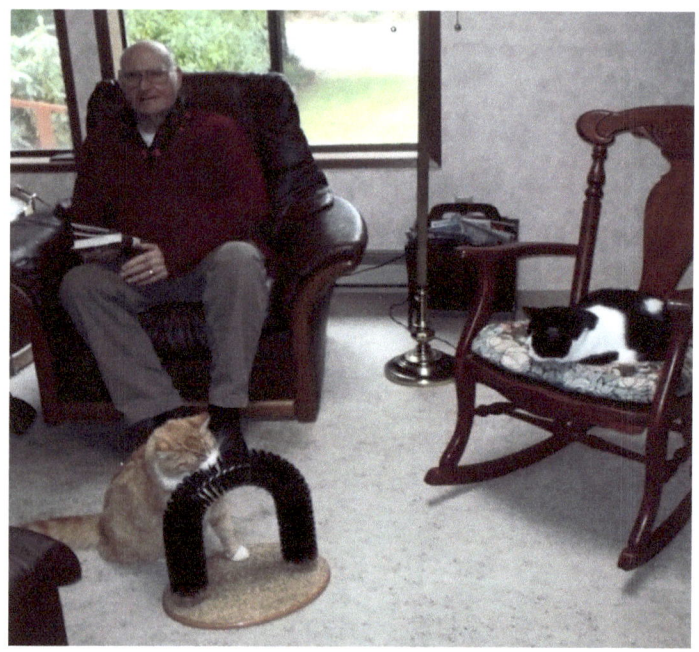

Enjoying an afternoon looking at pictures of airplanes gave Don pleasure. He was a private pilot and also loved cars, so both entertained him. I kept up subscriptions to golf, car and plane magazines for several years, then just kept magazines for he was unaware of having looked at the same ones over and over.

In our case I casually mentioned I thought we didn't need two vehicles any more while we were near the Ford dealership. And since we'd bought our SUV to pull a trailer that we'd sold, it was a plausible statement.

"Let's see how much this car is worth these days," I suggested. We pulled in where the car had been serviced for years, and eventually walked out with a check.

When the salesman offered too little it was I who said no, for Don saw this just as a lark, an interesting way to spend an hour or two. Back and forth we went, the salesman going in to talk with the boss about my disagreeing with his offer. By late afternoon a deal was struck, and whether my husband understood it was a lasting one at that time, I'm not sure.

For several years he was upset at his car being gone, sometimes quite upset. I countered his griping with what I hoped were soothing words, "We don't need two now. This car is like a sports car." It didn't quite do the trick, but I'd accomplished something that *had to be done*.

Another situation became our riding lawnmower. One spring it was obvious a serious accident could happen if he were driving. I wasn't sure how to handle the situation but I decided to get out the instructions and read them so I could use the machine.

"I'm going to jump on the mower," I said one day, heading for the garage. I can't remember how it went—maybe there were no repercussions or maybe Don mowed part. From that spring on, however, I encouraged him to come out with me.

"I need you to help me," I told him. He followed me around to the back yard, then, as I finished there, I motioned I was moving out to the front. After the mower was put away he joined me in using a broom to sweep the driveway, then, "Let's go in and have a nice cool drink."

Days varied, some being easier than others, and occasionally it was best if I set up a chair on the deck so he could watch from there rather than walk around the uneven yard. I made sure he had one of his favorite magazines in case he became bored.

When we don't see someone for a while their condition shocks us. One visit I've never forgotten is this: Before experiencing dementia in our own family we arrived to spend the night with friends who had stored a bit of furniture at their home while we traveled. That weekend we planned to remove it from their garage. As we sat at the table after dinner the phone rang and Dorothy reached for it. Just before hanging up I was aghast to hear her say, "Well, they seem to be taking everything. I don't know if they are going to leave us with even a bed to sleep in tonight." I'd known she had failed physically and mentally, but certainly not to that extent!

So if someone is going to visit after an extended absence, warn them of your loved one's disease. It will allow everyone to enjoy the visit without embarrassment or confusion.

CHAPTER SIX

Changes - Physical & Mental

As we age, our stomach, bowels, memory, speed, joints, all change. So it wasn't a great surprise when I found it necessary to begin each morning with MiraLAX for Don, mixed into a tall glass of cranberry juice. Constipation had been a recurrent problem for him, and this helped that as well as giving him the juice that may be most useful for healthy urination. To top it off, he loved cranberry juice. Don's stomach posed no problem, and he enjoyed all foods, including one of his favorites, liver. He gobbled up anything I put before him, like scrambled eggs with sausage, chopped apple, spinach, mushrooms and onions all mixed in. There were no cholesterol, diabetes, or high blood pressure foods to avoid. That may be a problem for your loved one, so be careful to take into consideration what the best diet may be.

We'd always enjoyed our coffee I'd mixed, half regular and half decaf; I continued that, though one cup at breakfast was all he wanted.

Steak, even cut up, became too difficult to chew up and swallow. So we changed to hamburger. Boiled chicken sausages were easy for him to eat unless the skin was thick, and I often skinned them after heating. If he acted like some food wasn't interesting, I grabbed the catsup bottle and added a dollop of that. Soon I saw a smile on his face.

Whole wheat bread had always been a favorite, and I made it a practice to give up all white bread, including hot dog and hamburger buns. Even sourdough bread I eliminated. The roughage in whole wheat was essential, I'd always believed. And I found rice to be constipating, so we seldom ate that as Don's disease progressed.

Eventually I began cutting up all his food and giving him a spoon for eating everything. I helped him eat some things, especially when he was tired. But he usually fed himself. *Being tired, though, made a big difference in a great many things, and it could be from a long day or sleeping poorly.*

Sleep apnea affects thousands and is described as a sleep disorder characterized by pauses in breathing or instances of shallow breathing while a person sleeps. Those pauses, called apnea, may last for a few seconds to several minutes. Five episodes an hour are necessary for a diagnosis. The abnormal shallow breathing is called hypopnea.

We knew people who wore the sleep apnea masks, but now the doctor recommended Don be tested. Many people give a loud snore or snort when they get back to normal breathing, but I'd never heard that from him. In a small room in our doctor's building he was hooked up with many sensors before going to sleep about 7:00 PM, then monitored throughout the night. His diagnosis was positive for that disease to the point it would cause cognitive changes.

There are many different types and sizes of masks, but he needs a full one that fits from forehead to chin. Medicare and our own insurance together cover the machine and mask, with delivery of new plastic masks, air hose and filters every few months.

After that he never slept without that valuable CPAP machine securely strapped over his nose. Don didn't mind the mask, but a person with claustrophobia might have trouble. One night all could be fine and the next night a hellish one of getting up and down to see why the mask was noisy or he was tugging at it.

Be sure extra supplies are available for changing, because a mask is plastic and becomes less soft and pliable as it ages. It must be washed and fit properly on the face or its use is worthless. There should be no sound except a steady, quiet breathing. If necessary, take the mask off and begin again. You should also inspect the entire mask to check that it's assembled correctly and all parts fit together securely. I occasionally found I hadn't pushed hard enough to click the pieces together.

A body slowing down after age 60 is normal, but disease of any kind may seem like it's running instead of walking. Don's appears to have progressed slower than some, but from month to month there were things I noticed.

Dressing himself was a gradual change. After having put on his own underwear and socks, he began being confused about it. I helped him with his slacks by having him sit on our bed and pulling them up at his own speed. But on days when he had trouble with dressing in general, I sometimes admonished, "You've done this every day, so why can't you do it this morning?" However, that obviously made no sense to him, for he'd stare at me and I'd realize my mistake. But the next day I might say the same thing. It took a while for me to understand he really needed help and wasn't just trying my patience. I was definitely a slow learner!

The same was true when it came to buttoning his shirt and pants, and zipping up his fly. However, tucking in his shirt before he buttoned his pants was automatic. Obviously it was a practice of so many years it was natural, but, I wondered, why weren't those other things? Dexterity played a part in it, of course. Eventually I ordered elastic waistband slacks and got rid of the others. So as abilities waned, I found I was dressing him completely. If he did something correctly, I praised him. I believe that is important. It may not mean he could remember how to do it the following day, but he felt good at the time.

When showers became merely standing under the water without using soap or washing his body, I began joining him. I started with his shampoo and worked down, always the same, so he knew what to expect. A washcloth nearby helped keep stinging shampoo out of his eyes. Baby shampoo which never stings, was recently suggested, but at the time I hadn't thought of it. At first he got out to dry off while I washed myself, but as with everything else, that became too much, so he stood beside me while I soaped up and rinsed. Then we both got out and I helped him dry his body. I loved to see him smile and took it for granted, but as most of us will discover, some days smiles are rare. Laughter is a wonderful experience, and seeing our loved ones losing that makes our lives dreary. I don't believe it means unhappiness as much as a part of the disease. It's hard to imagine a person with a humorous streak like Don could ever lose that. But little by little, he did. Occasionally when a cousin or old pal stopped by, or one of his kitties did something that tickled him, I saw it return.

Anything you can do to produce laughter will make a day brighter for you both.

One Christmas I ordered a set of DVDs of old Johnny Carson shows, and later a set of Dean Martin's programs. Both were funny and contained a lot of music, which he enjoyed. And he could *relate* to them; it wasn't just the music, and certainly not the jokes. *They were entertainers he remembered.* Often I put one of them on in the afternoon and heard or saw him guffawing. We both enjoyed it—he the funny acts, me his laughing. I-pods full of music make a day brighter, too.

Until recently I had never wondered about what Don *thought* he was saying in that jumbled speech, believing he was simply making noises because he couldn't pronounce words any longer—or know their meaning. I had humored him by saying, "Yes," or "sure" or "do you think so?"

But might he really be talking to me, unaware I couldn't understand what he was trying to say? Maybe he was asking, "Will you help me to the bathroom?" If I said, "Sure," and smiled, sitting there, unmoving, not understanding his question, it would be worrisome and confusing on his part. He would never know I didn't understand his words. *Why wasn't I taking him to the bathroom?* I began to watch for signs of this. Possibly it would help make life easier for him. And I asked the caregivers to do the same. Together we may have solved a piece of the puzzle for the time being.

We must never forget, however, that this disease is a progressive one, and what is true or may work one day, won't at some time in the future.

Enjoy everything you can along the way!!!

CHAPTER SEVEN

Wandering

To wander about the house at night or outside day or night is not uncommon. I hadn't considered it something I had to worry about until I got a phone call late one afternoon. Our golf pro had observed Don walking aimlessly a block from home and brought him back, only to find the house empty. I was out. So he knew it was important to phone me. I was shocked, and that was the last time I played poker on Thursday afternoons. I'd always turned the golf game on TV for him before I left. He'd seemed happy to see me home, but if he'd been out wandering I was unaware of it.

Getting up to roam around the house during the night never happened to us. One lady told me her mother attached a long scarf or piece of material from her wrist to her husband's and they slept that way.

I locked the front screen door on summer days and that prevented Don from going out without my knowledge. I went with him as he enjoyed walking down the driveway or in our cul-de-sac, but with a gravel road I knew I couldn't get him up if he fell. If you live in the country the situation is so different from the city where sidewalks make it easier to go for a stroll. But slipping or falling are bad wherever you might be.

Calling 911 for assistance after a fall can prevent you from straining or harming your bodies. If there's no injury you can explain it's not an emergency.

After I made the decision not to leave him alone, I noticed he wanted to be wherever I was continually. I told him when I was merely going into the next room, and if I went to the far end of our modest-sized house, I often turned around to find him behind me.

"You can stay here," I'd say. "I'll be back in a minute, as soon as I put this away." It seldom satisfied him, but it didn't matter. He felt better when he could see me. *I'd give anything now to turn around and see him up on his feet walking behind me. That's the reason I say to be grateful for whatever you have at the moment.*

We must try to live in the present and not worry about the future. Worry is detrimental and never produces anything positive!

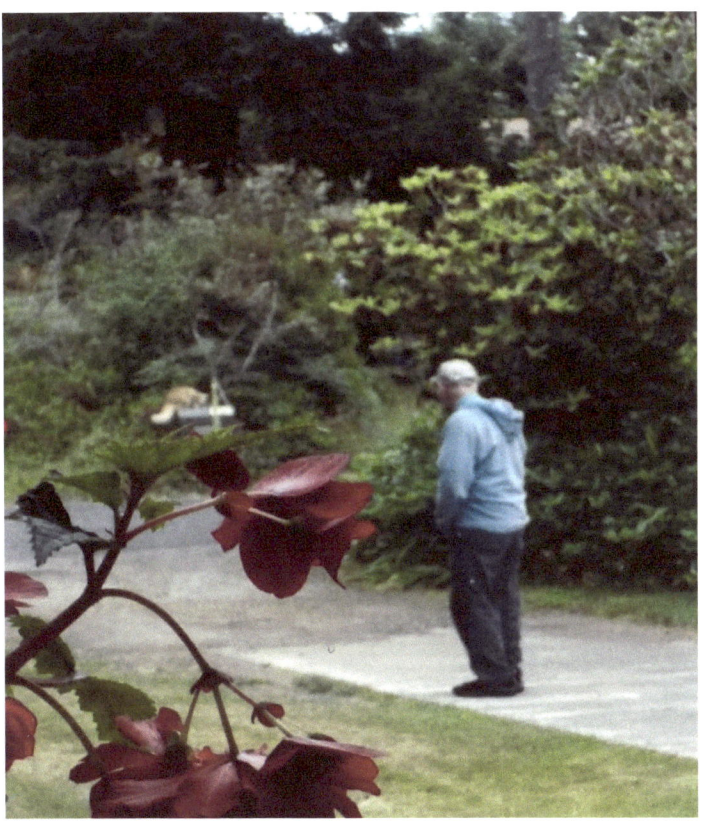

Sidewalks (if you have them) and driveways are the best places to walk, and it's obvious why in this photo. Living in a rural area means a companion should walk along when a loved one Is unsteady or is on gravel.

CHAPTER EIGHT

Alert Devices

I first ordered help alert bracelets for each of us when I felt Don might fall while walking his kitties. I explained the way he should push the button. At first I believed it was possible for him to understand, but soon I realized the bracelet would be for me if I were with him and we needed help. Since I have post-polio syndrome from having had polio when I was young, I was happy to have one for myself as I became less steady on my feet, and I put Don's away in a drawer. The range of ours was indoors, of course, but also in the yard for a certain distance. It also included one for travel, but every company may be different.

It may help you to feel more secure if the person understands the purpose of a bracelet or necklace (they come in both configurations). But if you have no need for one yourself and the walker who suffers from Alzheimer's or dementia can't understand, it's a waste of money. However, keep in mind, as conditions change or worsen, you may find it helpful—or you may want to get a cell phone.

Be sure to look into the cost and ways the devices work and differ. One may be more beneficial than another.

CHAPTER NINE

Memory Care & Paying for It

When you discover you cannot care for your loved one any longer, there are memory care facilities. They are expensive, and some are much, much better than others. Do a lot of searching before making your decision.
Look into what help you can get from state offices. I've added up the cost of in-home caregivers, and in most cases they are extremely expensive if you need round-the-clock help. In addition to paying them, you also have the cost of food, rent or mortgage, taxes, and many other expenses. So don't be in a hurry; look for what's best for your situation.

In the memory care home in which Don lived he shared a room with another man which was pleasant as well as saving money. Everything was included in his home, however, be extremely careful about add-ons. Just because a facility has a waiting list doesn't mean it's better than others. Read the reviews from people who have knowledge one way or another—carefully. **See last chapter of my additions.**

By all means, visit them or have a trusted friend or relative inspect any you are seriously considering. Observe the way they treat the people: are they caring; do they touch them by rubbing shoulders, or touching their heads and cheeks; do they smile at them? Their softness and obvious caring I believe is a testament to the entire little community. **Also see the last chapter.**

If you discover a family history of dementia of any type you should investigate *long-term care insurance*. It may help by paying part or all of the cost for assisted living or memory care—if the affected person qualifies. In one case I know of, however, a nurse came to the house to evaluate the one applying for assisted care. The husband, who was on oxygen and had difficulty getting around, qualified; the wife was well and knew she did not. She could live in the community with him but had to pay. When she became ill a year later, she also was eligible to live there free through their insurance. They moved from one assisted care facility to another to be nearer their children and that same qualification applied.

Since then I've heard of long-term care insurance running out after a certain number of years. And at one place the monthly statements of proof that were sent to the facility, cost $20 to fill out (with only a date change added) were raised to $40. This may be normal, but it's something to ask about.

There are many stories of people never qualifying after spending large sums for years to purchase the insurance. If you outlive that, it can't be helped, of course. It's a gamble. But if you have a history of poor health or family history of a disease that worries you, it is worthwhile to at least look into long term care insurance. Then you can make your decision wisely.

Veterans can get assistance paying for both assisted care and memory care, as expected. Contact the Veteran's Administration well in advance to see how this is handled.

If you choose to place the person you love into a memory care facility, don't feel you are giving up or shunning him or her. These homes welcome your visits; you make life happier for the people they are caring for.
But I made a huge mistake, believing what I'd been told, that you should allow the new resident to become acquainted with his home for two weeks before coming to visit. Now I can only imagine how lonesome and forlorn Don felt, hence his walk outdoors when he fell on the grass.

After being taken to the ER for that, another day he became dizzy and fell in the dining room, hitting his head with another trip to the ER. At some point during those two or three days his doctor started him on a huge dosage of Depakote for aggression, and whether that high dosage caused both of these falls I'm unsure, but I suspect so. Instead of beginning light, his doctor did the opposite. It happened during the time I was told I should stay away but *I should have been investigating and with him!*

Follow my words, not my example, for I was very, very wrong!

During the two years of his life in memory care I went in and helped Don eat breakfast, then wheeled him around the halls and out into the enclosed courtyard. Sometimes I pointed out the color of flowers, or counted the blossoms on a rose bush. One day we watched a gardener clip bushes, then blow the fallen twigs and leaves away. When an airplane flew over it was a special occasion. In the first home they got two cute little black kittens, and we watched them play.

Depending upon the level of comprehension, some residents color pictures, play with blocks, and do simple puzzles. Musical movies are popular, and soft music on the TV is often playing when no other activities are going on. The mind is soothed by music.

Memory care communities often have volunteers. At Don's the son of a resident played his guitar and sang for an hour at least once a week. A man whose wife once lived there came in several times a week to chat with the residents, wheel them around, walk or sit with them. I was always pleased to see my husband's instinct for friendliness still existed as he shook the volunteer's hand extended to him. Gus was a man who obviously enjoyed life and I found his enthusiasm for the men and women therapeutic for him as well as those who lived there. Dogs that are specially trained and licensed came to visit. They were very popular with the residents, and their happy faces were wonderful to see. On his better days Don kept time with the beat of the guitar music, and I was surprised to see him snap his fingers a time or two. Occasionally he teared up, and I attributed that to the fact his father played the guitar and banjo, so maybe that or a familiar song brought back memories. Also, crying doesn't always mean sadness in a dementia patient.

Some mornings those who were able sat in a semicircle with a huge balloon for balloon toss. A caregiver handed out long, colorful Styrofoam bats, and it became a wonderful game, even though some merely poked at the balloon; others who were well enough slammed it with great force. The purpose, of course, was to exercise their bodies.

I volunteered for many years at an assisted care home, helping with games; you might be welcomed to play the piano or some activity where you don't have to be a trained caregiver.

Caregivers are loving and patient and extremely kind. One told me, "I treat everyone here like they were my father or mother."

There's a number code I pressed for getting in and out the front door, and we were warned not to let anyone follow us either way.

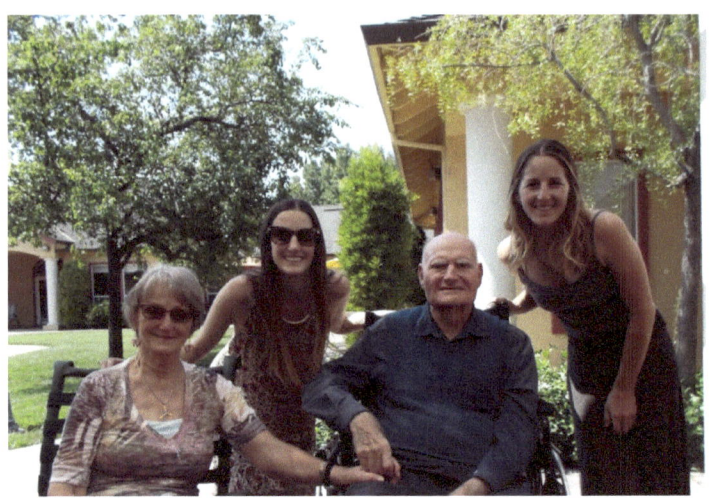

This picture of Don and me with our granddaughters was taken at his memory care home. The girls remember the times in our car many years ago when they sang songs with Grandpa at the top of their lungs. Our car was often alive with happy voices!

Behind us is the inner courtyard where residents can walk freely.

CHAPTER TEN

Caregivers & Agencies

The word "caregiver" includes a myriad of people—husbands, wives, friends, volunteer groups, and many paid males and females.

As a spouse, it's very hard to decide on the best way to handle day to day life when each duty is new to us in a way we haven't had to deal with before. For example, just brushing my husband's teeth could become a big squabble or a pleasant experience.

"Doesn't that feel good," I might say as I saw a grimace beginning. "Your teeth are sure looking good." Some days that worked and other times it didn't, or blew up into something worse.

     1—Always speak positively but firmly.
     2—After something is completed, say, "Good job!"
.   3—Explain what you want him or her to do, or you're going to do, beforehand, then see if they understand.

Friends offered to stay with Don, but I never said yes because he liked me to be with him. Being separated wasn't a thing I needed for myself. But if you long to get out and away, be sure to take those offers. In some cities there are groups who volunteer to stay with ill people. Of course it depends upon whether your loved one is easy to care for or not. I know of one ill person who refused someone coming in, though the spouse might have welcomed it.

THESE ARE IMPORTANT SOURCES OF INFORMATION:

In the rural area of Washington state where we lived, a friend with a disabled husband needed time to get away for errands and shopping.

She began by contacting **Senior Assistance** and was given the phone number for **Information and Assistance** for the county.

Then her name was given to the **Family Caregiver Support Program**. She and her husband were interviewed in their home and it was determined they were entitled to 32 hours a month (eight hours a week) of *respite care*.

Catholic Community Services was one of many different groups that serve the area, and they provided assistance. It took a while to get it all set up, but now she treasures the time she has free to do what is necessary.

In any area you can phone your county's **Senior Assistance** office and ask for help with *respite care*. You may need to follow up with another call, but stick to it!

When I was searching for a permanent memory care home for Don (as well as assisted care for myself) I was fortunate to be steered to a private entity, **Safe Senior Options.** The lady I spoke with visits the homes personally, so she can provide information firsthand. Those offices work with counties, hospitals, individuals like myself, and anyone who needs help. That service is free.

We've all heard of professional, licensed caregivers like **Visiting Angels, Caring, A Place for Mom, Elder Care**, and many more. You can look at their websites online and call them for information.

Take notes so you are able to spend time comparing them and see how they fit your needs: how they get to your home, cost per hour, food preparation, help with incontinence if necessary, and absolutely anything you want answered. No question should be off limits.
I was sent lists of homes from *Caring* and *A Place for Mom* over the internet when I searched for a memory care facility and assisted care home. You don't need to be online to get info; if you don't have a computer, phone them.

Support groups can be uplifting, spiritually helpful, and comforting. Talking about your problems and listening to solutions others have discovered or heard about, lessens your feeling of being alone. You may find neighborhood-sponsored get-togethers; there are also organized county and religious meetings, bi-monthly or monthly. So if you're interested, see if there are support groups in your community.

CHAPTER ELEVEN

Today — Our Lives

2017

As I look back over our life together I am so glad we took advantage of "living."

When times were tough in the mid 1980s Don found the forklift business in central California dying off, with farmers and businesses making do with what they had rather than buying new ones. And I discovered medical offices were changing—paperwork had become a headache, and the true medical work I'd always loved, waned.

One day we decided to sell everything and go see the United States in an RV, and for ten wonderful years we motored from one campground to another. Using that as a home base for a few days to several weeks, we explored the area in our tow car, a funny-looking little VW, called a Baja Bug. That was the start of our travels.

After we settled down we began traveling to countries in Europe with only backpacks for luggage. No reservations, no plan, just wandering. Few may think that sounds like fun, but we did, and that's what counts in life. Do what makes you happy and satisfied—both of you!

I encourage you to either think about things you want to do if you're young, or reminisce about what you've done. If it's the former, don't put off doing what thrills you. It doesn't have to be expensive if you're young—we were fifty years old when we began. But you probably will never regret a "wild and crazy" time, whether it be for a day, a few weeks, or many years.

Don is living in a memory care facility now, not far from my assisted care home, and I go to spend weekday mornings with him. Sometimes he merely looks at me when I arrive to help him eat breakfast, and other times he smiles. He always holds my hand, and I tell him how much I love him. His speech is garbled sounds usually, but occasionally I'm so happy to hear him say, "I love you."

I wheel him outdoors when there are no planned activities and I pull out the airplane magazine that's become tattered by its trips to him. "Look at that plane here," I tell him. "There's a red one. And here's a tail-dragger like you learned to fly in." He may be interested one day and fall asleep the next. Life is like that for him now and I have come to grips with it.

But what makes me feel happy through and through is what I experienced the other day. He'd been wheeled into the bathroom and I'd sat waiting for him, ready to go outside. When his caregivers returned, pushing him toward me, I saw his face become excited as he saw me. He waved his hands and was laughing by the time he was wheeled up beside me.

"He's sure happy to see you," one caregiver exclaimed.
I gave him a kiss through my tears of happiness. Life is very different and difficult now, but there are snippets of joy! And I'm so thankful for them.

ADDITIONAL COMMENTS

I have learned important things in the months since writing this book. Everyone's situation is different, but what I've discovered could affect a great many of you. It has to my loved one—and consequently me.

My first advice can't be more important or said enough times: as Power of Attorney you are the person who determines how your loved one is cared for. If you see something detrimental, contraindicated or unsafe, you are the one who can and <u>must</u> get it changed or discontinued.

After placing Don in the large, 50-person memory care facility, I began wondering if it had been my best decision after the following situation occurred. At Thanksgiving this past year I invited a friend to their luncheon, a lady whose husband is in a 6-person home after having had several strokes. When she was shocked at the noise and confusion, I was surprised at her disappointment. I wrote it off to her own situation and personality.

But now, after circumstances not of my making, I was forced to move Don. This time I chose a private home of 11 people after having looked into two smaller 6-person houses like the one of my friend's husband. That, for Don, I felt was too small, but for some it might have been fine—he'd always been a "people person."

A few questions were important to me when I placed Don in the first and now removed him from the second place:

Are the residents able to stay until the end of life, because I've learned some do not if they require too much care, even if they've said otherwise? <u>Not necessarily; if they require too much care, as they claimed in Don's first one, they must go to another home or a skilled nursing facility (SNF)</u>

Do they have a real interest in *good* care? <u>Not necessarily; if they require too much care, as they claimed in Don's first one, they must go to another home or a skilled nursing facility (SNF) .</u>

Were the caregivers able to put on a sleep apnea mask correctly? <u>No, none I've discovered have ever been trained in CPAP machines and have little interest.</u>

Would they encourage Don to do the things he was or should be able to handle? <u>Seldom.</u>

Is the room pleasant with a window? <u>So far, yes.</u>

The new home was considerably more expensive than where he'd been living, but after talking to the owner about what they offered and how they cared for their residents, I decided it was better than others I'd seen. I was unaware that small homes were more expensive.

To my surprise and anguish, I discovered **this new home was worse than I could ever have imagined**! For five weeks (while I looked for a new place) Don was never gotten out of bed while he languished in a room all by himself. Food was so poor that he lost 20 to 30 pounds in those weeks.

Finally, now in a Skilled Nursing Facility, run like a hospital, he's looked after with caring, smiles, dressed and in wheelchair. Physical and speech therapy are in-house. *One fee covers everything.*

Beware of occasional aides who have a mean streak. I reported one for trying to force Don's arms into positions that hurt him when trying to force them into shirt sleeve openings.

Be careful of add-on cost for needs. That may become more expensive than a one-fee-only home. And when past caring about where he /she lives, don't pay more for "pretty" places.

I asked his doctor to prescribe a mild sedative when Don was moved to a new home; but once settled the caregivers felt he needed more for he was noisy and nervous. Heavy medication had previously caused him to fall twice and become wheelchair-bound, but *his SAME doctor insisted on that SAME one instead of increasing* *the mild sedative.* *After a couple of days of sleeping all day I had to use my status as POA to get that cut in half; when he continued to mainly sleep I asked to have that lower dose restricted to bedtime only.* (Those words sound instructive but mild. In truth I argued vehemently with the doctor over the phone to get that dose cut. It was not what he wanted to do!)

When I'd fallen for the online quack several years ago and withdrawn Don's meds for about ten days early in his disease he was happier and able to speak more easily. Now I Googled to ask about discontinuing Aricept and Namenda. To my surprise my online information told about a type of dementia I'd never heard of, called FTD or frontotemporal degeneration (front of brain and sides, above the ears). Info of early symptoms of difficult speech and muscle rigidity jumped out at me because those were some of Don's first problems. For that Alzheimer's disease medications are not given. To see if that might be his correct diagnosis I requested the 2012 brain scan report by a neurologist in another state be looked at once more. *Had Don been misdiagnosed all along? He had not.*

To see if aggression diminished I asked, then demanded, Aricept and Namenda be discontinued. When he was more tranquil I did the same with the harsh, overpowering sedative to finally none at all. The change was heartwarming, and I always say, over and over, quality is more important than quantity!

At his former, large memory care home, without advance warning, I was told by the director that Don needed more care than they could give. Nothing had prepared me for that short, curt statement. I'd been about to go home for lunch that day and had a ride waiting, so through my tears I told her I had to go. At my assisted care home the manager gave me the phone number of the *ombudsman* that represented both homes. And she asked if I'd been given the *required written notice* from Don's residence, which I hadn't.

An ombudsman is an invaluable person. He or she is an advocate for you, one who knows rules and laws you probably don't. I asked for a meeting with them; so with the memory care home manager, their nurse, a visiting nurse, and my ombudsman, I met for over an hour. I spoke up when I heard statements I knew were untrue or disagreed with; there is no need to be aggressive, but do be firm and truthful.

After you've accomplished what you want with the ombudsman's help it might result in no action to a formal complaint. It depends upon the seriousness of the problem and your wishes. Don't let anyone intimidate you, but be careful not to let your emotions lead you into a bad situation. Talk over any concerns with the ombudsman.

Not having confidence in a doctor or wanting a second opinion is reasonable and if your physician objects that *would be a good reason to find another one, for* everyone has that lawful right. (I am in that process.)

Overmedication is another situation to be aware of, and since I've experienced this I've discovered it is a common problem. If your loved one shows unusual behavior, speak up. You will no doubt find yourself in difficult situations from time to time, but you owe your best to the one you care for. **See (C) above.**

Whether the person is in his own home or in memory care, **physical therapy may help in keeping muscles from becoming rigid.** If your doctor doesn't suggest it, ask him or her.

Keep good records, for when I recently worked on my income tax prep I was reminded how costly this disease is. If I hadn't been conscientious about saving all bills for housing, medications and other expenses, I wouldn't have been ready to prove them. You should ask the doctor for a statement explaining the reason for your loved one's special living arrangement or home care; keep this with your other papers in case of an audit.

We must be on guard constantly. That's the reason for this chapter. This terrible and sad disease is a constant learning experience I've found over and over.

ADDITIONAL COMMENTS, TWO

My dear husband passed away on March 21, 2018, and as I sat down to write an obituary for his hometown paper in Paris, IL and our weekly newspaper in Washington, I got the date of death wrong. That hard-to-imagine error revealed my confusion and sense of loss. While I was relieved he wasn't suffering any longer the shock of losing him was evident. Don's life had been what my son and I had called "a zero" for many months.

After years of watching the devastating nature of his illness I've voiced my opinion of life many times: **quality is more important than quantity**. That firm belief evolved as I watched the deterioration of spirit, humor, abilities, and finally recognition of people.

For the past two years each weekday morning I'd left my assisted living apartment, eager to see Don. I became anxious to get down the long hallway, always hoping to experience his smile when he saw me, the highlight of my day. One morning I'll never forget, I walked into his 4-bed room just as he was being readied for the activity room. He saw me and his eyes sparkled as a huge grin enveloped his face! At times like that it's hard to realize it may never happen again; and in fact, it never did, so spontaneous and loving and happy. That was about six months before the end, and something I think about often now. I find it makes me teary-eyed, yet it is heartwarming to reminisce about important milestones.

But little by little Don's wakefulness ebbed, and one of the last times I fed him applesauce or cookies he fell asleep before finishing. I knew the cause—his brain that had been in the process of being destroyed, had progressed significantly.

Here is a scientific description from the Alzheimer's Association: **Alzheimer's disease leads to nerve cell death and tissue loss throughout the brain. Over time, the brain shrinks dramatically, affecting nearly all its functions.**

After I tore the meniscus of my right knee at home in WA I believed if I had it repaired I'd be away from Don for some weeks. For that reason I decided to let it go, using a cane or walker to get around. The idea of taking time away from him for up to perhaps six weeks was something I felt I couldn't do, or didn't want to do. But fate is fickle, for the last five weeks of Don's life I was away. A severe virus struck me, leaving me coughing so severely and feeling so weak I could barely get from bed to chair to bathroom.

By the time I returned I found him on oxygen, and that night I got a call to come to his bedside. My family picked me up and we stayed with him until he appeared sleepy. Then we each gave him a kiss and left. As many have told me, at the end a patient often becomes more aware; that night Don's eyes gazed into mine as he lay in bed, and when I kissed him he kissed me back—both new occurrences.

As we left a nurse explained I could initiate Hospice contact—not caregivers in a nursing home or private residence. She would make the call so I could speak to a nearby Hospice office in the morning. I had known nothing about the procedure, and it turned out to be most fortunate for both Don and myself. The next day I came as usual, made that phone call, and stayed for lunch; an hour later a Hospice nurse and Social Service member arrived (and stayed with me). After I signed papers as Don's POA (Power of Attorney) morphine from the nursing home pharmacy was dripped into Don's mouth. His breathing, which had been fast and labored, quieted, and within an hour his eyes closed for a nap. I left, planning to return in the morning.

But during the night I received another call. Don had passed away at 3:40 AM. Because we had both willed our bodies to the nearby medical school, it was important I see him right away so his body could be moved within four hours. To my surprise a kind, loving Hospice nurse welcomed my daughter-in-law and me and gave me a big hug. In the middle of the night, I thought! How thoughtful could that be! She led us into Don's room, and as I kissed him I found his lips cold. I reached for his also-cold hand and held it as if I could warm it. *He had left his body and gone to a better place. It was a relief as well as one of forlorn loss to me.*

As we left she put Don's wedding ring on my right hand and patted it. Hospice is a compassionate organization (and it sounds cold to call such a group an organization, but of course it is a very large one.) She walked with us to the front door and reminded me to call if there was *anything* they could do to help. (They phoned me twice later to ask if I wanted help.)

Maureen and I found an open fast-food shop and got something to take back to my apartment. It was something I needed—company for talking. We spent an hour together, then she left and I began with a shower, getting ready for the day.

An amazing sight came to me, as clear as anything I have ever seen. Up toward the ceiling I saw very—extremely—clearly a white triangle, the Father, Son and Holy Ghost. I will never forget the moment and often try to see it again, but I believe that sight was sent to me only once, for reassurance and love. Since then I've felt Don's presence near me throughout the days and nights. It's a great comfort.

If your loved one's body is to go to a mortuary (which you probably will have made arrangements for as the end drew near), that call will begin a series of steps for you. But in my case, having no mortuary involved because his body was picked up and treated in a specialized way as all medical schools do, I had to do them myself.

HERE IS WHAT GOES ON, BY YOU OR THE MORTUARY:

(1) The **Death Certificate** is the most important.
If it's up to you, you (or a family member can help you) go online to **VitalChek.com** and fill out a form to order one or

more copies of the death certificate. My cost for one certificate was $52. It may take several weeks to receive.

   (1-a) As soon as possible call your loved one's insurance companies—including drug plan, banks, Medicare, Social Security, and any company involved.

   (1-b) When the death certificate arrives, immediately send *copies* to those insurance companies, banks, etc. From some you'll get a refund for what time is left and was paid for.

(2) If your loved one was married, it is important to set up an appointment with **Social Security** as soon as possible.

   (2-a) Call and find out what they need from you. **(see below)**

   (2-b) You can go to the Social Security **office** or get it done by **phone**, but you must get an *exact time* they will call you. Or if an appointment, be *sure to be on time*.

   (2-c) If the deceased was married, a spouse will not get both Social Security checks but the one which is larger. If a former divorced or deceased spouse had a larger Social Security payment than the one who just passed away, the remaining marriage partner is eligible for that one. In my case I made the choice to collect Don's though it was smaller. I was asked a second time, but it was my decision.

(2-d) For your *visit* to Social Security you must have: SS number of the deceased and your own; original death certificate; marriage license; any former marriage license (or date of marriage if that's all that's possible); divorce info (if possible); dates of birth of any children under 18; maiden name of wife and of all parents; *place* of birth of deceased and spouse; *date* of birth of both. If a **phone** call is your choice, you must *mail the original death certificate* to Social Security office, which will be returned.

(2-e) Finally you will tell SS where to send your check, or bank account numbers.

(2-f) To finish the visit or call you will write or vow that you've told the truth, which, during the phone call will be explained that it is like your signature.

Some answers are absolutely necessary and others they let pass. Be honest if you don't know and can't find out, but try to have all the information before the time of visit or phone call. It will take a few weeks before the change is seen on your account. Don't hesitate to ask questions; the SS person will answer them gladly.

Having a pet as well as loving family and friends I find invaluable. Tom, a cat I inherited two years ago, is my wonderful confidant, pal, and 12-year-old sounding board. At night when he cuddles up with me in bed, I tell him how I couldn't live without him. Every so often he'll reach out a paw to me. I know he's saying, "I understand, Anne, and

I'm so happy to be your best pal." If he could smile I'm sure it would be a huge one!

We must be on guard constantly. That's the reason for this chapter. This terrible and sad disease is a constant learning experience I've found over and over. I have good reason to report one of Don's doctors to the Medical Society, and am in the process of that now. I've done more fighting since becoming a POA than in my entire over-eighty years, but every Alzheimer's and dementia patient deserves the best we can provide.

When Treatment is Dangerous

In the last section I told you I was about to take punitive action, and now I have begun a chapter in my life as a Power of Attorney, that sadly, involves Don's life as a patient. Because my husband was given a medication so devastating to him, that he never again walked on strong legs, but became wheelchair-bound, I've made that decision.

If you are a POA for your loved one, don't hesitate to report injustice. In my case it changed a life dramatically, but it isn't always that stark.

First, get your facts from the perpetrator, be it doctor, owner of a home for the disabled, etc. If a doctor won't give you the entire information, as in my case, that may be serious enough to cause him grave problems.

Next, write a letter to the office that oversees the type of case you have; in my case it was the Medical Board of my state, but it could be a nurse, physical therapist, nursing home, or anyone who cares for people. If you aren't sure, ask questions or with a computer, Google your query to find out where to send your report. But don't be put off by anyone who downplays your concerns. Your loved one is fortunate to have you looking out for him or her.

In my case I sent a first complaint, then, after getting a letter back, I tried to get specifics from the doctor who overmedicated Don, but my request was refused. So I told the Medical Society about that and they told me, in language I could readily understand, *they could get it! And they did.*

Remember, stand up for what your POA was meant to be! You would want the same for yourself if necessary. You will never be sorry—in fact, you should be proud.

We must be on guard constantly. That's the reason for this chapter.
This terrible and sad disease is a constant learning experience I've found over and over.

I wish you all well! I want to thank those who helped me: Nancy Gorsche, a lobbyist in the 1980s, and Gail Garrard, a friend and writer, who edited many pages. Our loving family and friends have been the comfort I've need. Thank you all.   Anne

www.ingramcontent.com/pod-product-compliance
Lightning Source LLC
Chambersburg PA
CBHW040322220526
45473CB00009B/2532